CHAIR PILATES FOR SENIORS OVER 60

10 Minutes Daily Exercises for Beginners To Lose Weight And Improve Mobility, Strength And Balance

Randy T. Lucas

Table of contents

INTRODUCTION

Meet Jessica, a vibrant 63-year-old who exudes youthful energy despite the occasional reminders of her body's age. She embarked on a quest to revitalize her spirit and nurture her physical health, stumbling upon Chair Pilates, a practice that would transform her life.

As Jessica delved into Chair Pilates, something magical happened. She found a sanctuary in its gentle movements and empowering postures, a pathway to reclaiming vitality, strength, and flexibility.

Through Jessica's journey, the profound benefits of Chair Pilates for seniors over 60 became crystal clear. It's not merely a series of exercises; it's a lifeline to wellness, a conduit to a more fulfilling life.

This guide seeks to encapsulate Jessica's experience, offering a roadmap to rejuvenation, vitality, and enhanced well-being for seniors exploring Chair Pilates. Discover a tailored blend of seated exercises, mindful breathing, and fluid movements designed specifically for the unique needs of individuals over 60.

In the chapters ahead, we'll uncover the secrets of Chair Pilates, understanding its principles, exploring custom exercises, and embracing a holistic approach that goes beyond physical fitness to include mental clarity and emotional balance.

Are you ready to embark on a journey that breaks the shackles of age, offering a path to a more vibrant and fulfilling life? Let's dive into the world of Chair Pilates for seniors over 60 together.

CHAPTER 1

Understanding Chair Pilates

Chair Pilates is a modified form of the traditional Pilates exercise system, tailored to accommodate the needs of individuals with limited mobility or those who prefer a seated workout routine. Rooted in the core principles of Pilates, this practice aims to improve physical fitness, flexibility, core strength, and overall well-being, making it particularly suitable for seniors over 60.

At its core, Chair Pilates revolves around controlled, deliberate movements that focus on engaging specific muscle groups while seated. The primary goal is to develop a strong and stable core, enhance flexibility, and improve posture. Utilizing a chair for support and stability, participants can perform a wide range of exercises that effectively target various muscle groups.

Breathing techniques are fundamental in Chair Pilates. Mindful and controlled breathing is synchronized with movements, facilitating better oxygen flow throughout the body, enhancing relaxation, and promoting focus during exercises.

The practice places a significant emphasis on alignment, precision, and fluidity of movement. Even though the exercises are performed in a seated position, they effectively engage the core muscles, including the abdominals, back, hips, and shoulders. This engagement helps in building strength, improving stability, and supporting better posture, which is particularly beneficial for seniors aiming to prevent falls and maintain balance.

Chair Pilates exercises are gentle and low-impact, making them accessible to a wide range of individuals, including those recovering from injuries or dealing with physical limitations. The adaptability and versatility of Chair Pilates routines enable participants to customize workouts based on their fitness levels, gradually increasing intensity and complexity as they progress.

Moreover, the practice's emphasis on controlled movements and mindful breathing not only nurtures physical health but also contributes to mental well-being. Chair Pilates serves as an avenue for stress relief, promoting relaxation, mental clarity, and overall emotional balance.

In essence, Chair Pilates offers a holistic approach to fitness and wellness for seniors over 60, providing a gentle yet effective means to improve strength, flexibility, balance, and mental focus while seated in a supportive environment.

Benefits for Seniors Over 60

1. Improved Flexibility: Chair Pilates exercises promote flexibility, aiding in joint mobility and reducing stiffness commonly associated with aging.

2. Enhanced Core Strength: Engaging core muscles in seated movements helps strengthen the abdominal and back muscles, improving stability and balance.

3. Better Posture: Practicing Chair Pilates can correct and maintain proper posture, reducing strain on the spine and enhancing overall body alignment.

4. Increased Muscle Tone: Regular practice helps tone muscles, preventing muscle atrophy and maintaining muscle mass.

5. Joint Health: Gentle movements in Chair Pilates support joint health by lubricating and strengthening the joints, reducing discomfort and enhancing mobility.

6. Improved Balance and Coordination: Chair Pilates exercises aid in enhancing balance and coordination, reducing the risk of falls and injuries.

7. Stress Reduction: Mindful breathing techniques incorporated in Chair Pilates can help alleviate stress and promote relaxation.

8. Boosted Energy Levels: Engaging in Chair Pilates regularly can increase energy levels and overall vitality.

9. Enhanced Mental Clarity: The focus on mindful movements and breathing can improve mental focus and clarity.

10. Customizable Workouts: Chair Pilate's routines can be tailored to individual needs and abilities, accommodating varying fitness levels and specific health conditions.

CHAPTER 2

Getting Started

Safety precautions and guidelines for practicing Chair Pilates

1. Consult with a Healthcare Professional: Before starting any exercise program, especially if you have pre-existing health conditions or concerns, consult with your doctor or a qualified healthcare professional to ensure Chair Pilates is suitable for you.

2. Use a Stable Chair: Ensure the chair you use for Chair Pilates is sturdy, stable, and has a solid backrest to provide adequate support during exercises.

3. Check for Proper Alignment: Sit in the middle of the chair with feet flat on the floor, knees aligned with hips, and maintaining a straight back to ensure proper posture during exercises.

4. Start Slowly and Gradually: Begin with gentle movements and exercises, gradually increasing intensity and complexity over time to avoid overexertion or strain.

5. Listen to Your Body: Pay attention to your body's signals. If you feel pain, discomfort, or dizziness during any exercise, stop immediately and seek guidance from a certified instructor or healthcare professional.

6. Breathing Awareness: Focus on controlled breathing throughout the exercises, inhaling deeply through the nose and exhaling slowly through the mouth to enhance relaxation and oxygen flow.

7. Avoid Overextension: Perform movements within your comfortable range of motion without overextending or pushing beyond your limits to prevent injury.

8. Proper Form is Key: Concentrate on maintaining proper form and alignment during exercises, emphasizing quality over quantity to maximize benefits and reduce the risk of strain.

9. Hydration and Rest: Stay hydrated before, during, and after the session. Take breaks when needed and allow your body adequate time to rest and recover between exercises.

10. Gradual Progression: As you become more comfortable with Chair Pilates, gradually incorporate new movements and increase the duration or intensity of exercises, allowing your body to adapt progressively.

Adhering to these safety precautions and guidelines will help ensure a safe and enjoyable Chair Pilates experience, minimizing the risk of injury while maximizing the benefits for seniors over 60.

Choosing the Right Chair and Setup

Choosing the appropriate chair and arranging the setup for Chair Pilates is crucial to ensure safety, stability, and effective practice, especially for seniors over 60. Here's a guide on selecting the right chair and arranging the setup:

1. Sturdy and Stable Chair: Opt for a chair that is sturdy and stable, preferably without wheels, to prevent any unexpected movement during exercises. A chair with a solid, flat seat and a strong backrest provides better support.

2. Comfortable Seat Height: Ensure the chair's seat height allows your feet to rest comfortably flat on the floor, with knees bent at a 90-degree angle and hips level with or slightly higher than the knees when seated.

3. Solid Back Support: The chair should offer adequate back support. If needed, you can place a small cushion or a rolled towel behind your lower back for additional support and to maintain proper spinal alignment.

4. No Armrests or Adjustable Armrests: Ideally, choose a chair without armrests or with adjustable armrests that can be moved out of the way during exercises to allow for better movement and freedom.

5. Non-Slip Surface: Ensure the chair's surface is non-slip to prevent any accidental sliding or movement while performing exercises.

Setup:

1. Clear Space Around the Chair: Create a clear and spacious area around the chair to ensure freedom of movement during exercises. Remove any potential hazards or obstacles that might hinder your movements.

2. Positioning: Place the chair on a flat and even surface, ensuring it's positioned in a way that allows you to move your arms and legs comfortably without hitting nearby furniture or walls.

3. Good Lighting and Ventilation: Choose a well-lit and ventilated space for your Chair Pilates practice to enhance comfort and safety.

4. Personalization: Customize your setup based on individual needs. For instance, if you need additional support, consider using props like pillows or yoga blocks to modify exercises for comfort and safety.

By selecting an appropriate chair and arranging a suitable setup, seniors over 60 can ensure a safe, comfortable, and effective Chair Pilates practice that maximizes the benefits of the exercises while minimizing the risk of injury.

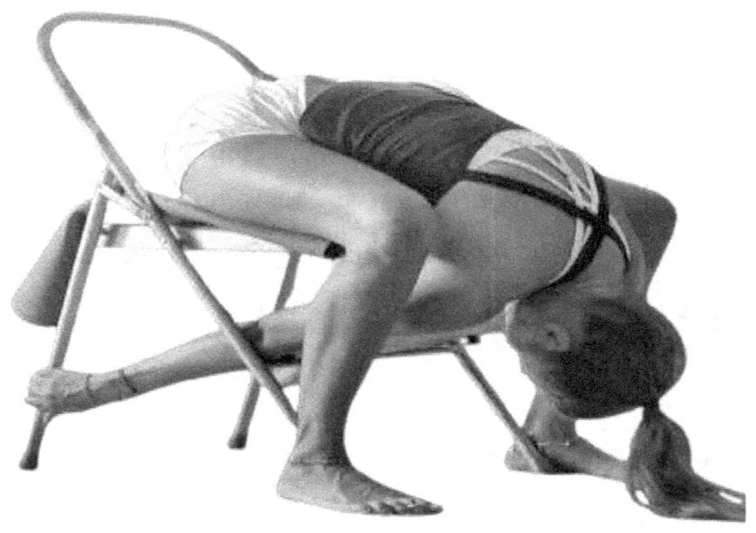

CHAPTER 3

Basic Chair Pilates Exercises

Breathing Techniques:

1. Diaphragmatic Breathing:

Sit comfortably with your feet flat on the floor and hands resting gently on your abdomen. Inhale deeply through your nose, allowing your abdomen to rise and expand. Exhale slowly through youGr mouth, contracting your abdomen inward. Repeat this deep breathing pattern for several breaths, focusing on the rise and fall of your abdomen.

2. Pursed Lip Breathing:

Sit upright and inhale deeply through your nose. Exhale slowly through pursed lips, as if blowing out a candle, while slightly contracting your abdominal muscles. This controlled exhalation helps to regulate breathing and promote relaxation.

3. Segmented Breathing:

Sit comfortably and slowly inhale through your nose, dividing the breath into three equal parts - first filling the lower lungs, then the middle, and finally the upper lungs. Exhale slowly in the reverse order, releasing the air from the upper, middle, and then lower lungs. This technique helps in maximizing lung capacity and mindful breathing.

4. Counted Breathing:

Sit quietly and inhale deeply through your nose, counting to four. Hold the breath for a count of four, then exhale slowly through your mouth, counting to four again. Repeat this cycle, focusing on maintaining even and controlled breath counts.

5. Alternate Nostril Breathing (Pranayama):

Sit comfortably and place your right thumb on your right nostril, inhale deeply through the left nostril. Close the left nostril with your ring finger and release the right nostril, exhaling through it. Inhale through the right nostril, close it with the thumb, and exhale through the left. Repeat this cycle, focusing on slow, controlled breaths through each nostril alternately.

These breathing exercises are designed to promote relaxation, improve lung capacity, and enhance mindfulness, serving as an essential foundation for Chair Pilates practice for seniors over 60.

Seated Warm-Up Movements:

1. Shoulder Rolls:

Sit comfortably with your feet flat on the floor. Relax your arms by your sides. Lift your shoulders up towards your ears, then roll them back and down in a circular motion. Perform gentle shoulder rolls, aiming for a smooth and controlled movement. Start with 8-10 rolls in one direction, then switch to the opposite direction.

2. Head Nods:

Sit tall and relax your shoulders. Gently nod your head forward, bringing your chin towards your chest, and then slowly lift your head back to a neutral position. Repeat this movement for 8-10 repetitions, focusing on the stretch in the back of your neck.

3. Arm Circles:

Sit with your feet flat on the floor and extend your arms out to the sides at shoulder height. Make small circular motions with your arms, rotating forward for 8-10 repetitions, then reverse the direction for another 8-10 repetitions. This exercise helps loosen up the shoulders and improve mobility.

4. Ankle Circles:

Sit with your feet flat on the floor and extend one leg forward. Rotate your ankle in a circular motion, first clockwise for 8-10 repetitions, then counterclockwise for 8-10 repetitions. Switch to the other leg and repeat. This movement helps in improving ankle flexibility and mobility.

5. Seated Cat-Cow Stretch:

Sit on the edge of the chair, place your hands on your knees, and inhale as you arch your back, lifting your chest and tilting your pelvis forward (Cow). Exhale as you round your spine, tucking your chin towards your chest, and bringing your belly button towards your spine (Cat). Repeat this gentle cat-cow movement for 6-8 cycles, synchronizing breath with movement.

These seated warm-up movements are gentle yet effective in preparing the body for Chair Pilates exercises, enhancing mobility, flexibility, and circulation for seniors over 60.

Core Strengthening Exercises:

1. Seated Marching:

Sit upright at the edge of the chair, engage your core muscles, and lift one knee toward your chest while keeping the other foot firmly planted on the floor. Alternate legs in a marching motion, focusing on maintaining stability and engaging your abdominal muscles. Aim for 10-12 marches on each leg.

2. Seated Leg Extensions:

Place your feet level on the ground and sit tall. Stretch one leg forward and hold it there for a few seconds while maintaining it parallel to the ground. Return the leg to its starting position slowly. Continue with the opposite leg. For each leg, do 8–10 repetitions, paying close attention to using your core to stay balanced.

3. Seated Side Bends:

Sit with your feet flat on the floor and arms extended overhead. Inhale and lengthen your spine. Exhale as you bend to one side, sliding your hand down the chair's side. Inhale back to the center, then exhale and repeat on the other side. Perform 6-8 repetitions on each side, engaging the core to stabilize your body.

4. Seated Torso Rotation:

Sit tall and hold the sides of the chair with both hands. Exhale as you rotate your torso to the right, twisting from the waist and looking over your right shoulder. Inhale back to the center and repeat on the left side. Perform 6-8 rotations on each side, focusing on controlled movement and engaging the core.

5. Seated Pelvic Tilts:

Sit with your feet flat on the floor, and place your hands on your hips. Inhale and tilt your pelvis forward, arching your lower back slightly. Exhale and tilt your pelvis backward, rounding your lower back. Repeat this gentle pelvic tilt movement for 8-10 repetitions, focusing on engaging the core muscles.

These core-strengthening exercises in Chair Pilates aim to engage and strengthen the abdominal muscles, improve stability, and support better posture for seniors over 60.

CHAPTER 4

Intermediate Chair Pilates Exercises

Gentle Stretching and Flexibility Movements:

1. Seated Forward Fold:

Sit at the edge of the chair, feet flat on the floor. Inhale, lengthen your spine, then exhale as you hinge at the hips, folding forward from your waist. Hold for 15-20 seconds, feeling a gentle stretch in your lower back and hamstrings. Return slowly to an upright position.

2. Seated Side Stretch:

Sit tall and reach your right arm overhead, gently leaning to the left, feeling a stretch along the right side of your torso.

Hold for 15-20 seconds, then switch sides, reaching the left arm overhead and leaning to the right.

3. Seated Spinal Twist:

Sit tall with feet flat on the floor. Twist your upper body to the right, placing your left hand on the outside of your right thigh and your right hand on the back of the chair for support. Hold the twist for 15-20 seconds, then switch sides.

4. Seated Hip Opener:

Sit tall and cross your right ankle over your left knee, allowing your right knee to gently fall open. Keep your back straight and lean forward slightly, feeling a stretch in your right hip. Hold for 15-20 seconds, then switch legs.

5. Seated Shoulder Stretch:

Sit tall and extend your right arm across your chest. Use your left hand to gently press the right arm towards your body, feeling a stretch in the right shoulder. Hold for 15-20 seconds, then switch arms.

6. Seated Hamstring Stretch:

Extend your right leg forward, heel on the floor, and flex your foot. Keeping your back straight, lean forward slightly, feeling a stretch in the back of your right leg. Hold for 15-20 seconds, then switch legs.

7. Seated Cat-Cow Stretch:

Sit on the edge of the chair with feet flat on the floor. Inhale as you arch your back (Cow), then exhale and round your spine (Cat). Repeat this gentle cat-cow movement, synchronizing breath with movement for 6-8 cycles.

Balance and Coordination Exercises:

1. Single Leg Balance:

Sit upright and lift one foot off the floor, extending the leg forward. Hold the position for 10-15 seconds, engaging your core for balance. Switch to the other leg and repeat.

2. Chair Squats:

Stand in front of the chair with feet hip-width apart. Lower yourself towards the chair as if sitting down, then return to standing position without fully sitting. Repeat this squatting motion for 10-12 repetitions, focusing on controlled movement and using the chair for support if needed.

3. Heel-to-Toe Balance:

Stand behind the chair, holding it for support. Step one foot straight ahead of the other, heel to toe. Try to maintain this position for 15-20 seconds, then switch feet.

4. Leg Swings:

Holding onto the chair for balance, swing one leg forward and backward, keeping it straight. Perform 10-12 swings on each leg, controlling the movement and engaging the core for stability.

5. Seated Leg Cross and Uncross:

Sit tall and cross one leg over the other. Then, uncross and cross the other leg on top. Alternate crossing and uncrossing the legs for 8-10 repetitions, engaging the core and maintaining balance while switching legs.

6. Side Leg Lifts:

Stand beside the chair and hold onto it for support. Lift one leg out to the side, keeping it straight and engaging your core. Lower it back down slowly. Perform 8-10 lifts on each side, focusing on controlled movement.

7. Standing Calf Raises:

Stand behind the chair with feet hip-width apart. Rise up onto the balls of your feet, lifting your heels as high as possible, then lower them back down. Perform 10-12 calf raises, engaging your calf muscles and using the chair for support if needed.

These intermediate Chair Pilates exercises offer a variety of gentle stretching movements and balance-focused exercises, aiming to enhance flexibility, stability, and coordination for seniors over 60.

CHAPTER 5

Advanced Chair Pilates Moves

Building Strength and Endurance:

1. Seated Leg Lifts:

Sit tall at the edge of the chair, engage your core, and lift both legs straight out in front of you. Hold for a few seconds, then slowly lower them back down without touching the floor. Aim for 8-10 repetitions, gradually increasing as you build strength.

2. Seated Knee Tucks:

Sit with your knees bent and feet flat on the floor. Lean back slightly, engage your abdominal muscles, and lift both knees towards your chest. Hold for a moment, then extend your legs back out. Perform 8-10 repetitions, focusing on controlled movement.

3. Seated Side Leg Extensions:

Sit tall and extend one leg out to the side, keeping it straight. Lift the leg upward, then slowly lower it back down without touching the floor. Perform 8-10 lifts on each leg, engaging the outer thigh muscles for strength.

4. Seated Triceps Dips:

Sit at the edge of the chair with your hands gripping the edge beside your hips. Lift your body off the chair, bending your elbows and lowering your hips toward the floor. Push back up to the starting position. Aim for 8-10 dips, focusing on using your arm muscles to lift your body weight.

5. Seated Russian Twists:

Sit tall, lean back slightly, and lift your feet off the floor, balancing on your sit bones. Hold your hands together and twist your torso to the right, then to the left, touching the floor beside your hips with your hands. Perform 8-10 twists on each side, engaging your core throughout the movement.

6. Seated Leg Circles:

Sit tall on the chair with your hands holding the sides for support. Extend one leg straight out in front of you. Circle the leg clockwise for 5 repetitions, then reverse the direction for another 5 repetitions. Switch legs and repeat, engaging the core and hip muscles.

7. Seated Bicycle Crunches:

Sit at the edge of the chair, lean back slightly, and lift both feet off the floor. Bring one knee towards your chest while extending the opposite leg straight out, then switch sides in a pedaling motion. Aim for 8-10 alternating bicycle crunches, focusing on engaging the abdominal muscles.

Progressing Safely in Difficulty Levels:

1. Chair Push-Ups:

Stand facing the chair, place your hands on the edge of the seat, and step your feet back to an angle that challenges you. Lower your chest towards the chair by bending your elbows, then push back up to the starting position. Aim for 8-10 push-ups, adjusting the difficulty by changing the angle of your body.

2. Single Leg Stand:

Stand behind the chair and lift one leg off the floor, balancing on the other leg. Hold this position for 15-20 seconds, then switch legs. Increase the challenge by extending the time and maintaining balance.

3. Standing Knee Lifts:

Holding onto the chair for support, lift one knee towards your chest, then extend the leg straight out in front of you. Return to the starting position and repeat on the other side. Perform 8-10 lifts on each leg, focusing on controlled movement and balance.

4. Standing Leg Swings:

Stand beside the chair and hold onto it for support. Swing one leg forward and backward, keeping it straight. Perform 10-12 swings on each leg, controlling the movement and engaging the core for stability.

5. Standing Heel Raises:

Stand behind the chair with feet hip-width apart. Rise up onto the balls of your feet, lifting your heels as high as possible, then lower them back down. Perform 10-12 calf raises, engaging your calf muscles and using the chair for support if needed.

6. Chair Plank:

Stand facing the chair, place your hands on the seat, and step your feet back into a plank position. Keep your body in a straight line from head to heels, engaging your core muscles. Hold the plank position for 15-20 seconds, gradually increasing the duration as you build strength.

7. Standing Leg Balance with Arm Reach:

Stand beside the chair and lift one leg off the floor, balancing on the other leg. Simultaneously, reach the opposite arm up and overhead, lengthening through the body. Hold for 10-15 seconds, then switch sides, focusing on stability and controlled movement.

These advanced Chair Pilates exercises are designed to challenge strength, endurance, and stability for seniors over 60, while also providing a safe progression in difficulty levels.

CHAPTER 6

Modifications and Adaptations

Tailoring Exercises for Individual Needs:

1. Chair Height Adjustments: Adapt exercises by modifying the chair's height. For individuals with limited mobility or flexibility, using a higher chair or placing cushions on the seat can reduce the distance to the floor, making exercises more accessible.

2. Range of Motion Modifications: Tailor exercises to accommodate varying ranges of motion. Individuals with limited mobility can perform smaller movements initially, gradually increasing as flexibility improves. For example, reduce the leg lift height or arm extension range.

3. Use of Props: Incorporate props like resistance bands, small weights, or pillows to assist or challenge movements based on individual abilities. For instance, using a resistance band for added support during leg exercises or holding a small weight during arm movements can modify intensity.

4. Seated versus Standing Variations: Modify exercises by allowing individuals to perform movements in a seated or standing position, based on their comfort and stability. Those with balance concerns may benefit from seated variations while gradually progressing to standing as confidence improves.

Addressing Common Challenges:

1. Joint Pain or Stiffness: Adapt exercises by focusing on gentle movements that avoid excessive strain on joints. Encourage individuals to perform slow and controlled motions, emphasizing comfort and avoiding pain triggers.

2. Balance Issues: Modify exercises to include the use of a chair or nearby support for stability. Incorporate seated exercises initially, gradually progressing to standing exercises with the support of a stable surface or chair as needed.

3. Muscle Weakness: Tailor exercises to target specific muscle groups while gradually increasing resistance or repetitions. Start with low-intensity movements and progress slowly to build strength without causing strain.

4. Fatigue or Limited Endurance: Adapt routines by allowing for adequate rest between exercises and gradually increasing exercise duration or intensity over time. Encourage participants to listen to their bodies and take breaks as needed.

5. Breathing Challenges: Modify breathing techniques by practicing shorter durations initially and gradually extending breath counts as lung capacity improves. Encourage individuals to focus on comfortable breathing patterns.

These modifications and adaptations in Chair Pilates empower seniors over 60 to personalize their practice, addressing individual needs and overcoming common challenges while ensuring a safe and effective exercise regimen.

CHAPTER 7

Chair Pilates Routines

Sample Daily, Weekly, and Monthly Routines:

Daily Routine (Approximately 10-20 minutes):

1. Warm-Up (3 minutes): Start with gentle warm-up movements, such as neck rolls, shoulder rolls, seated marches, and spinal twists, to prepare the body for exercise.

2. Strength and Flexibility (5 minutes): Perform a mix of strength-building exercises like seated leg lifts, arm circles, and core-engaging movements like seated knee tucks or side leg extensions. Include gentle stretching exercises like forward folds or side stretches for flexibility.

3. Balance and Coordination (3 minutes): Incorporate balance-focused exercises such as single-leg stands, leg swings, or standing heel raises to enhance stability and coordination.

Weekly Routine (Approximately 3-4 sessions per week):

Variety and Progression (30-40 minutes per session): Focus on different aspects of Chair Pilates in each session. For instance, dedicate one session to core strengthening exercises, another to flexibility and stretching, and another to balance and coordination. Gradually increase exercise intensity or duration as endurance improves.

Monthly Routine (1-2 sessions per month for longer, more intensive workouts):

Intensive Workout (45-60 minutes per session):

Use these sessions for a comprehensive workout. Include a mix of all elements - warm-up, strength-building exercises, flexibility stretches, balance-focused movements, and perhaps introduce new, slightly more challenging exercises to keep the routine engaging and progressive.

Customizing Routines for Varied Abilities:

1. **Individual Assessments:** Conduct individual assessments to determine participants' abilities, limitations, and preferences. Tailor routines based on their fitness levels, mobility, and specific goals.

2. Progression and Modification: Gradually progress routines by increasing repetitions, intensity, or complexity as individuals improve. Conversely, modify exercises by offering seated variations, reducing range of motion, or providing additional support as needed.

3. Personalized Approach: Encourage participants to mix and match exercises based on their comfort and needs. Allow flexibility in choosing routines to accommodate preferences while ensuring a well-rounded workout.

4. Incorporate Rest and Recovery: Emphasize the importance of rest and recovery between sessions. Encourage participants to listen to their bodies and take breaks when necessary to prevent overexertion.

Customizing Chair Pilates routines allows seniors over 60 to adapt their workouts to their abilities, ensuring a safe, enjoyable, and effective exercise regimen that caters to individual needs and goals.

CONCLUSION

In embracing Chair Pilates, seniors over 60 embark on a journey not just toward physical fitness but also toward holistic well-being and vitality. As we conclude this guide, it's evident that Chair Pilates transcends mere exercise: it becomes a doorway to a more enriched and vibrant life.

Throughout this journey, we've uncovered the remarkable benefits that Chair Pilates offers to the senior community. From the gentle yet effective movements to the profound impacts on strength, flexibility, balance, and mental clarity, Chair Pilates emerges as a fountain of rejuvenation and resilience.

Chair Pilates is not about achieving unattainable feats or pushing the limits beyond comfort; rather, it's about embracing progression at one's own pace. It stands as an embodiment of adaptability, allowing each individual to tailor their practice to suit their unique abilities, preferences, and challenges.

Moreover, this practice extends beyond the physical realm. It serves as a sanctuary, nurturing mental resilience, instilling confidence, and fostering a sense of inner harmony. The focused breathing techniques, mindful movements, and gentle stretches not only strengthen the body but also nourish the spirit, fostering a profound connection between body, mind, and soul.

As we part ways, let us carry forward the wisdom garnered from Chair Pilates—its adaptability, its profound impact on well-being, and its testament to the enduring strength of the human spirit. Let this practice not just be a part of a routine but a steadfast companion in the journey toward a more vibrant, fulfilling, and resilient life.

May Chair Pilates continue to serve as a beacon of hope, resilience, and vitality for seniors over 60, guiding them toward a life brimming with joy, strength, and an enduring sense of well-being. Let us embrace the legacy of Chair Pilates as a testament to the beauty of aging gracefully and living life to the fullest.

FITNESS

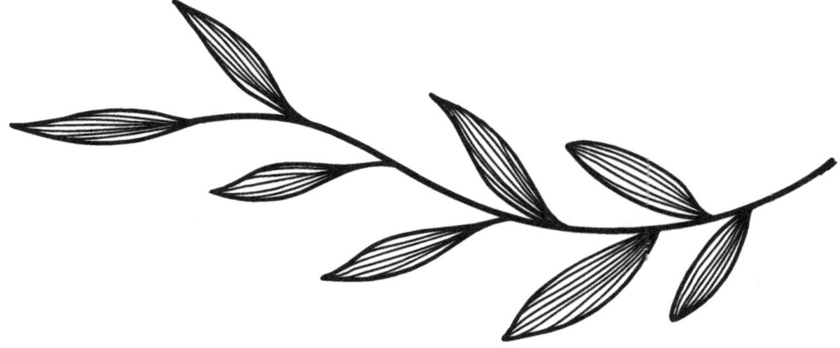

PLANNER

Fitness Planner

NAME: **DATE:**

BREAKFAST

LUNCH

DINNER

SNACK

EXERCISE   SET   REP   NOTES

Fitness Planner

NAME: **DATE:**

BREAKFAST

LUNCH

DINNER

SNACK

EXERCISE

EXERCISE	SET	REP	NOTES

Fitness Planner

NAME: **DATE:**

BREAKFAST

LUNCH

DINNER

SNACK

EXERCISE

SET	REP	NOTES

Fitness Planner

NAME: **DATE:**

BREAKFAST

LUNCH

DINNER

SNACK

EXERCISE   SET   REP   NOTES

Fitness Planner

NAME: **DATE:**

BREAKFAST

LUNCH

DINNER

SNACK

EXERCISE

SET	REP	NOTES

Fitness Planner

NAME: **DATE:**

BREAKFAST

LUNCH

DINNER

SNACK

EXERCISE

SET	REP	NOTES

Fitness Planner

NAME: **DATE:**

BREAKFAST

LUNCH

DINNER

SNACK

EXERCISE   SET   REP   NOTES

Fitness Planner

NAME: **DATE:**

BREAKFAST

LUNCH

DINNER

SNACK

EXERCISE

SET	REP	NOTES

Fitness Planner

NAME: **DATE:**

BREAKFAST   LUNCH

DINNER   SNACK

EXERCISE   SET   REP   NOTES

Fitness Planner

NAME: **DATE:**

BREAKFAST

LUNCH

DINNER

SNACK

EXERCISE   SET   REP   NOTES